My Back Hurts!

Handbook for Seniors with Back Pain

by Orthopaedic Surgeons

Richard J. Nasca M.D. and James D. Hundley M.D.

Illustrations by Madeline White

Previous Book in the **MyBones** Series

My Hip Hurts! Causes and Treatments of Hip Pain in Seniors
2018

Coming soon in the **MyBones** Series

My Knee Hurts! Handbook for Seniors with Knee Pain

My Neck Hurts! Handbook for Seniors with Neck Pain

MyBones Publishing Company
via Amazon CreateSpace, 2018

Introduction

This is the second in the **MyBones** series of condition-specific books for non-physicians authored by board certified orthopaedic surgeons. Each book focuses on a specific area: neck, back, hip, knee, shoulder, elbow, hand, ankle and foot along with several other topics that could be helpful to you. Please search on Amazon.com from time to time to see if a **MyBones** book addressing your area of concern has become available.

Medical science is complicated. When doctors talk, we use language foreign to most people, even those highly educated in other disciplines. Intelligent people want to understand their medical problems. We hope that this booklet will provide you and your loved ones a better understanding of your diagnosis and treatment options.

Two seasoned orthopaedic surgeons combine over 100 years of training and experience to help demystify the language of their profession. Moreover, they offer opinions on how they would wish their loved ones and themselves to be treated.

We believe this information will help you better communicate with your physician and will enable you to ask relevant questions to get useful answers. We want you to avoid problems when possible and take an active role in helping your surgeon determine the best course to follow when help is needed.

Our training after university consisted of four years of medical school followed by five years of specialized training in orthopaedic surgery under intense supervision. After two years in the U.S. Navy, one went into academic surgery where he practiced orthopaedic surgery and trained future surgeons. After two years as an orthopaedic surgeon in the U.S. Air Force, the other joined a group of orthopaedic surgeons in private practice.

We take full responsibility for what we say, but please remember that we are expressing our opinions based on training and experience. Medical science changes rapidly, so what seems to be true today may not be so tomorrow. Furthermore, it is common for medical people to have different opinions, so your surgeon may have opinions different from ours. We are telling you what we think and believe to be true.

Reading this booklet does not make one an expert in the field. It cannot take the place of professional, in-person consultation. If your condition is persistent or worsening or you need more specific information about your case, please see an orthopaedic surgeon as soon as possible.

Be enlightened! Be empowered! Be healthy!

Table of Contents and Overview

Chapter 1: Spine Anatomy

In order to understand the diseases and disorders that occur in the back, namely the lumbar and thoracic spine, a review of spine anatomy and commonly used terms is provided.

Chapter 2: Commonly Used Imaging and Other Tests

Several imaging studies and tests are used to evaluate spine disorders and diseases.

Chapter 3: Non-Surgical Options of Back Care

Various medications, injections, physical therapy, bracing and pain management are discussed.

Chapter 4: Common Disorders Affecting the Back

Herniated disc, slipped vertebra, spinal stenosis, spinal deformity and sacroiliac (SI) joint dysfunction occur frequently and may require surgical treatment.

Chapter 5: Arthritis, Cancer of the Spine, Spine Infections and Spine Fractures

Many types of arthritis can affect the spine. Lung, breast and prostate cancer may spread to the spine. Other types of cancer like multiple myeloma may originate in the spine. In order to treat infections of the spine, antibiotics coupled with surgical treatment are often needed. Compression fractures due to osteoporosis are common in women following menopause.

Chapter 6: Complications of Spine Surgery

Surgical complications and the measures taken to avoid them are discussed.

Chapter 7: What to Expect after Spine Surgery

Better outcomes in spine surgery have occurred in the last decade due to better diagnostic techniques, less invasive procedures and better implants and instrumentation.

Glossary

Medical terms and phrases are defined to help you better understand the conditions and treatments discussed.

Acknowledgements

We appreciate those who have inspired and helped us in this undertaking.

About the Authors

Reviewer Comments

Chapter 1: Spine Anatomy

In order to understand the abnormalities that can occur in your spine, it is helpful to first understand normal spine anatomy and terminology.

The spinal column is made up of thirty-three (33) vertebrae joined together by very strong ligaments and the intervertebral discs. There are seven (7) cervical, twelve (12) thoracic and five (5) lumbar vertebrae. The five (5) sacral vertebrae form a single block of bone and are not joined together with intervertebral discs as are the other vertebrae. The coccygeal vertebrae are small and considered remnants of a tail.

When you are standing, you will notice that your cervical spine has a gentle inward curve which positions your head over your shoulders. This is referred to as a *lordotic* curve. The thoracic spine has an outward curve, which is referred to as a *kyphotic* curve. The lumbar spine has a lordotic curve. A spine lacking these normal curves is unable to provide normal posture and balance.

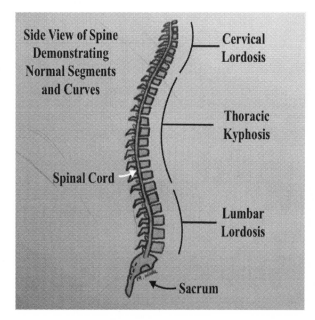

The sacrum is attached to the pelvic bone, the *ilium,* at the *sacroiliac joint.* The sacrum is angled backward from the fifth lumbar vertebra, the *lumbosacral joint.* The normal spine aligns the head over the pelvis and hips.

Each vertebra is made up of a cylinder of bone, *vertebral body*, arches, *pedicles*, and a roof like coverings, *laminae*, with an attached *spinous process*. These bony structures support, encase and protect the spinal cord and its nerves in the *spinal canal*.

The spinal nerves exit the *spinal canal* through windows called *foramen* located between vertebrae. Upper and lower projections called *facets* provide for attachment points between vertebrae as do the intervertebral discs which are composed of soft gelatinous interiors, *the nucleus,* supported by strong interlacing ligaments, the *annulus fibrosus*.

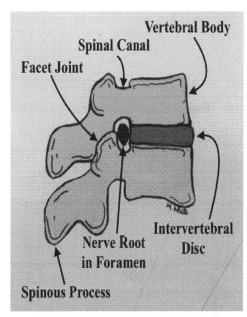

Side View of Spine Segment

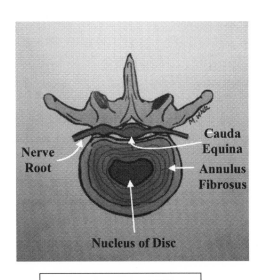

**Intervertebral Disc
Cross-section View**

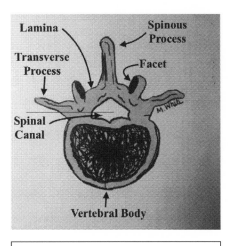

**Vertebral Body
Cross-section View**

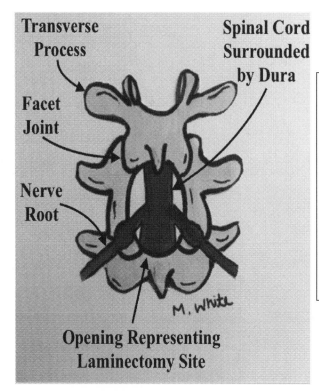

Transverse Process

Facet Joint

Nerve Root

Spinal Cord Surrounded by Dura

M. White

Opening Representing Laminectomy Site

Back view of spine segment with laminae removed, *laminectomy site*, showing dura covering spinal cord and exiting nerve roots

The cervical spine is attached to the base of the skull with very firm and strong ligaments. It is the most flexible part of the spine making it the most vulnerable to injury. The thoracic spine is the most rigid and least flexible part of the spine supported by twelve (12) ribs on each side. The lumbar spine is surrounded by large groups of muscles which enable us to maintain an upright posture and provide strength to our core.

Chapter 2: Commonly Used Imaging and Other Studies.

Spine surgeons rely on several types of imaging studies to guide them when making a diagnosis and planning treatment. Commonly performed X-Rays of the spine include front, side and oblique views. Standing views of the spine are commonly done to evaluate scoliosis and other spinal deformities. Bending films are useful in determining displacements of vertebra, unstable areas and flexibility of a spinal deformity such as scoliosis.

Bone scans are done by injecting a small amount of radioactive material into the patient. A scan of the skeleton is done to detect areas of abnormal accumulation of the radioactive material, which occurs in patients with infections, tumors and fractures.

In order to evaluate your bone density measurement, a DEXA, dual energy x-ray absorption, scan using low dose X-ray beams is done. A **T score** shows the amount of bone you have compared with a young adult of the same gender with optimal bone mass. A T score above -1 is considered normal. A T-score between -1 and -2.5 is classified as **osteopenia** (often called "thin bones"). A T-score below -2.5 is defined as **osteoporosis** (often called "soft bones" or fragile bones, high risk for fractures from minimal trauma).

Computerized tomography, CT scan, computer modulated x-rays, allow visualization of the spine in three dimensions. CT scans can be done rapidly and are most helpful in evaluating patients with spinal fractures and tumors. They are often done after the introduction of dye into the fluid surrounding the spinal cord and nerves, *myelogram,* to visualize these structures.

In contrast to CT scans, Magnetic Resonance Imaging, MRI, uses high strength electromagnets rather than radiation to image the spine. These studies provide a great deal of useful information in making a diagnosis and planning treatment. The MRI provides excellent visualization of bone and soft tissues such as ligaments, discs and neural structures from the front, side and along the cross-sectional planes of the spine. CT and MRI are used in surgery to guide the surgeon and to verify placement of implants and instrumentation.

Electromyography, EMG, detects abnormal nerve and muscle function by sampling the response of various muscles and nerves to signals from the brain. Nerve Conduction tests are used to evaluate whether or not a nerve stimulated by electricity transmits these signals and at what speed.

The function of the spinal cord and nerves is monitored by Somatosensory Evoked Potentials, SSEP, and Motor Evoked Potentials, MEP, during the various surgical procedures used to decompress, correct and stabilize the spine.

Various blood tests are of value in evaluating patients with spine complaints. These include tests for infection, sedimentation rate, white blood count, blood cultures, bone and tissue samples. Patients with arthritis are tested for rheumatoid factor, antinuclear antibody, lupus, gout, and other specific disease indicators found in the blood. Samples of spinal fluid are analyzed for cells indicative of infection, tumor or trauma.

Chapter 3. Non-Surgical Options in Back Care

Prior to considering any surgical procedure it is wise to pursue appropriate non-surgical therapy. Most surgeons recommend a three to six month course of conservative, non-surgical, treatments prior to spine surgery.

John, a forty-year-old accountant, awakes on Monday morning with a sore lower back following a weekend of doing yard work which included shoveling, digging and raking. He has a hard time getting out of bed. Bending over is painful due to spasm of the large muscles in his low back. Most likely, John has strained the muscles and ligaments, which support the vertebrae in his back. A few days of rest, ice packs and over-the-counter medication such as Motrin®, Aleve® and Tylenol® will in most cases resolve the problem. Stretching prior to doing yard work and using good body mechanics may have prevented his sore back.

It is estimated that during one's lifetime, most people will have one or more episodes of lower back pain. Often, these occur without any antecedent cause. As with John, who had a sedentary job, the cause of his acute back pain was probably due to his "not being in shape" to tackle the rigors of a weekend of yard work.

If your back pain causes you difficulty with your normal activities, what can you do to aid your recovery?

Following an acute injury to your back, ice applied to the painful area can reduce swelling and pain. Short periods of bed rest and a reduction in stressful physical activity may accelerate recovery. Corsets and elastic fabric braces may also be useful.

Non-steroidal anti-inflammatories drugs, NSAIDs, are often effective in reducing back pain and improving motion and function. Ibuprofen, naproxen and diclofenac are effective in alleviating inflammatory conditions of the spine joints and ligaments. Although serious side effects are rare, gastrointestinal bleeding, fluid retention, kidney damage and cardiac failure may occur with the use of **high** and **prolonged** doses of NSAIDs. Some **topical anti-inflammatories** by prescription are available and effective. Narcotics such as codeine, hydrocodone and oxycodone may be used for short term pain control following injury and surgery. Long term use results in dependence and addiction. Muscle relaxants may be of some value in the early phases of acute back and neck pain to reduce muscle spasms. Neurontin®, Gabapentin® and Tramadol® may also be useful.

Cortisone was discovered by Phillip Hench and Edward Kendall of the Mayo Clinic when they noted that during pregnancy some patients with rheumatoid arthritis got better and several went into remission. This was due to higher than normal levels of cortisol produced during pregnancy. In the late 1940s, cortisone became available. Short courses of oral steroids such as Prednisone® and Medrol® can be very effective in reducing nerve root and inflammation-generated pain. However, these medications do not result in any reversal of the arthritic process, which continues on.

Injection of various types of cortisone with local anesthetics into inflamed and arthritic joints has brought relief to many patients by disrupting the inflammatory cycle of pain. Patients with suspected infection and those on anticoagulants are not candidates for these types of injections. If needed, these injections can be given every four to six months.

Platelet Rich Plasma (PRP) collected from the patient's blood and stem cells harvested from fat and bone marrow injected into painful joints of the spine have been shown to reduce pain and improve function. These biologic approaches to treating back pain are gaining popularity. Long-term results from this type of treatment are not available.

Epidural steroid injections (ESI) are placed into the spinal canal outside the protective dura, the sheath surrounding the spinal cord and its nerves, to reduce nerve root generated pain. Several types of targeted nerve root blocks are used to determine which nerves are responsible for generating the pain in the cervical and lumbar spine. After injection of a local anesthetic, patients are asked if their usual pain is less or abated. The addition of cortisone to the diagnostic block may reduce the nerve generated pain for variable periods of time. These diagnostic nerve root blocks done by skilled physicians specializing in Pain Management using X-Ray guidance are extremely helpful in directing surgical treatment to the exact anatomical areas responsible for the patient's pain. For facet joint mediated pain, anesthetic blocks are done of the small nerves that supply these joints. If the patient has relief of pain, there are techniques to interrupt the nerve supply, *ablation*, to the painful joints.

Transcutaneous electrical nerve stimulators, TENS, are sometimes helpful in overriding and masking painful stimuli. These devices are applied to the skin around the painful area and the intensity and frequency of the current is adjusted by the patient. A device called a *dorsal column stimulator* can be helpful in managing patients with chronic pain due to various spinal disorders and following spinal surgery. The dorsal column stimulator is placed through a small incision into the spinal canal on the back surface of the dura. The generator is attached to the stimulator wires and is tested for effectiveness in reducing pain prior to its permanent implantation in the body. Pain Management physicians provide care for patients requiring further pain control with medications and injections following surgery.

Physical and occupational therapy can be effective in treating acute and chronic back pain. Stretching, strength training and supportive bracing under the supervision of a skilled therapist can be very helpful during the acute onset of a painful spine condition as well as during rehabilitation following surgery and trauma. Traction applied to the back is often helpful in relieving pain. Traction can be applied by using weights and pulleys or by machines. The zero-gravity inversion bed was popularized at the Sister Kenny Institute in

Minneapolis. It takes gravitational pressure off the nerve roots and discs of your spine, essentially "stretching the spine." If your joints are not taken to their limits on a regular basis, the amount of motion they will allow will diminish. We all lose some range of motion as we age, but we can counteract that somewhat and even improve our range of motion through stretching. Muscle strength training is important if you want to maintain function and agility in performing your routine daily activities without overloading and fatiguing the muscles that control the movement and alignment of your spine. Often the core muscles of the abdomen get lazy and need reinforcement by doing abdominal strengthening exercises such as bringing the knees up to the chest, tilting the pelvis toward your navel and doing sit-ups with your knees flexed.

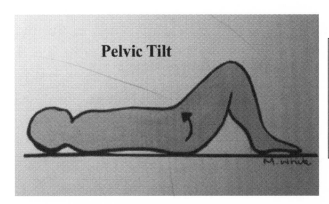

Lying supine and rotating the pelvis toward the abdomen into a pelvic tilt

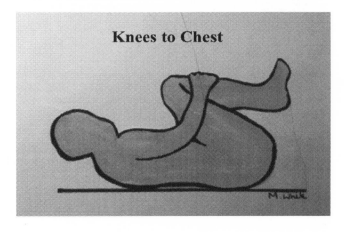

Lying supine and bringing the knees up to the chest

Sit-up starting from a supine position

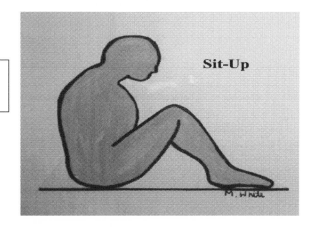

Several years ago, Robin McKenzie of New Zealand found that patients suffering acute back pain where more comfortable lying prone with their head and upper trunk elevated while waiting for him to treat them, McKenzie developed a program of extension-based spine exercises which if done on a regular basis improved the patient's extensor spine muscle strength and their ability to stand more erect and balanced. When an acute back attack occurs, one can try a prone position with elevation of the upper trunk on cushions to relieve pain and spasm in the low back area.

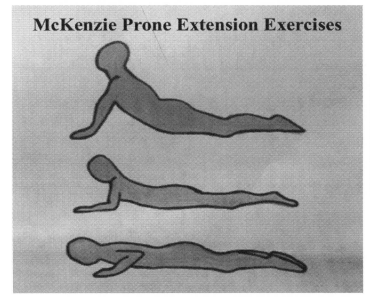

McKenzie Prone Extension Exercises

Prone extension exercises with gradual extension supported by forearms and shoulders

Lifting the head and upper trunk off the cushions against gravity with the arms while keeping the lower spine still will provide further relief.

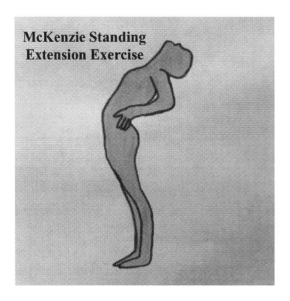

Many have likely been to chiropractors for back care. Many of these practitioners are well trained in providing non-operative care. Be sure you have had an adequate evaluation and diagnosis before undergoing treatment. We recommend seeing a medical doctor spine specialist if you have neurologic symptoms such as loss of feeling or weakness in your arms or legs or if your pain persists despite chiropractic treatment.

Chapter 4: Common Disorders Affecting the Back

Patients with back disorders usually complain of pain in the lower back which limits their mobility and interferes with their activities of daily living such as bending, lifting, dressing and sleeping. Spasms of the back muscles and referred pain into one or both lower extremities are common. Pain may radiate into the hip, knee or foot. It may be intermittent, sharp, dull or feel like pins and needles. If examination of the hip, knee and foot is normal, the physician should refocus on the spine.

Your doctor will ask you several questions about your complaints, then perform a physical examination with you standing, while checking your alignment and level of your pelvis. If your pelvis is not level, your leg lengths are measured. Your examiner will check for tender areas around the spinous processes, your range of motion both in flexion, extension and side bending and for spasms of your back muscles. Testing of your deep tendon reflexes, muscle strength and sensation in the lower extremities is done to determine any deficit in nerve function. Pulses in your legs are evaluated for blood flow and your abdomen probed for abnormal, *enlarged organs*, or pulsatile masses, *aneurysms*. On occasion, a rectal examination is needed to evaluate rectal tone after a spinal injury and in patients with a painful coccyx, *coccydynia*.

Herniated Lumbar Disc, Ruptured Disc

David, a 35-year-old attorney and avid golfer had acute pain in his low back and right leg after his Saturday morning round of golf. He had felt some twinges of pain during the round but kept playing. David tried to get back to work on Monday but he had to stay home because of severe leg pain and trouble walking because of weakness in his right foot. He was seen by an orthopedic surgeon, who after a brief examination, determined that David had a ruptured, *herniated disc*. The herniated disc was causing pressure on his fifth lumbar nerve resulting in weakness of the leg muscles that control the

19

upward movement of the ankle and foot during walking referred to as a "dropped foot." David was given medication for pain and a short course of oral Prednisone, which relieved some of his pain. MRI confirmed that he did indeed have a herniated disc, which was quite large and pressing on the nerve. He was given injections of cortisone in his low back and physical therapy, but he continued to have severe right leg pain and the dropped foot for which he underwent surgery. The surgeon removed a large fragment of disc material that had compressed his fifth lumbar nerve. Following surgery, he improved and returned to work.

The discs between the vertebrae function to provide motion and flexibility to the spinal column. As we age, the internal contents of the disc, the *nucleus,* loses hydration and structure. The outer casing of the disc, the *annulus fibrosus*, which supports the nucleus and binds the disc to the adjacent vertebrae, also loses structure and develops gaps called *fissures* though which the nuclear material can escape.

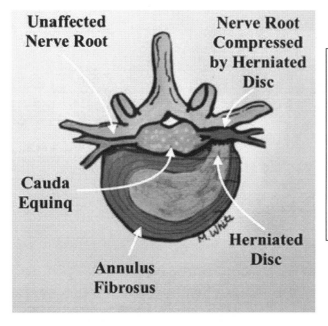

Unaffected Nerve Root

Nerve Root Compressed by Herniated Disc

Cauda Equinq

Annulus Fibrosus

Herniated Disc

Cross section of spine showing disc material herniated though a defect in the annulus resulting in compression of the nerve root

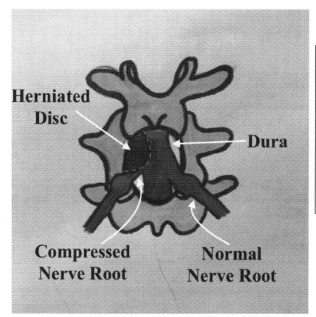

Herniated Disc

Dura

Compressed Nerve Root

Normal Nerve Root

View from the back of the spine with laminae removed showing a herniated disc compressing the dura and nerve root

When one applies torsion and compression to the spine as with the golf swing, the interlacing fibers of the annulus may separate and tear allowing the nucleus to herniate out into the spinal canal and encroach on the nerve root. If the nerve root is irritated but not physically compressed, pain without weakness will occur in the affected extremity. David had twinges of pain as he compressed and torqued his lumbar spine during the golf swing. He experienced the severe leg pain and the dropped foot when the disc material herniated through a defect in the annulus fibrosus and resulted in pressure on his fifth lumbar nerve root.

Each nerve root supplies innervation to different muscles. The level of disc herniation compressing the nerve root determines the muscle function disrupted. If the disc herniation occurs between the third and fourth lumbar vertebrae, the L4 nerve root is compressed resulting in weakness of the quadriceps muscle resulting in pain around the inside of the knee. Disc herniation between the fifth lumbar and first sacral vertebrae causes weakness of the foot and ankle muscles making it difficult for patients to walk on their toes.

If there is no neurologic deficit or bowel or bladder control issues, in most cases the back and leg complaints resolve within a period of three to six weeks. Loss of bowel or bladder control requires immediate surgical attention to remove pressure on the spinal cord or its terminal portion, the *cauda equina.* A progressive loss of muscle strength is another indication for surgical intervention.

MRI has been extremely helpful in visualizing the extent of the herniation and the resultant nerve compression. Patients with cardiac pacemakers cannot undergo MRI, so they may need to have a myelogram and CT scan. This procedure consists of injecting a water-soluble contrast agent into the spinal fluid and taking a series of x-rays followed by a CT scan.

Surgery to remove a herniated disc is a commonly performed and successful procedure requiring a day or less in the hospital or ambulatory center. A small incision is centered over the level of the herniated disc. A portion of lamina is removed to gain access to the spinal canal and affected nerve root. After carefully separating and protecting the nerve root from the herniated disc, the latter is removed. Prior to closing the incision, the surgeon will check to be sure there are no additional disc fragments and that the affected nerve root is free and mobile. Most patients experience immediate pain relief. Those with sedentary jobs can return to work within a few weeks. It is wise to limit lifting and return to sports for three to four months until there is healing of the annulus with scar tissue. Complications are rare. The most common are recurrent disc herniation, usually through the same defect in the annulus in eight to ten percent of patients and tears of the dura, which are repaired during surgery. **Lumbar Disc Replacement** may be an option in young patients with single level disc disease following surgery for herniated disc and for degenerative disc disease.

Slipped Vertebra, Spondylolisthesis

Jim, a fifty-year-old mechanic, had injured his fifth lumbar and first sacral vertebrae while playing tackle on his high school football team. He improved following treatment with a brace, physical therapy and medication. However, as the years went on, he continued to experience recurrent episodes of low back, hip, leg and foot pain. Standing for long periods and bending over caused increasing pain. Some days he was unable to carry out his job as an auto mechanic because of the back and leg pain. He took several types of over-the-counter medications to get through his workday. He got some relief from a back brace and chiropractic manipulation. An examination and a series of X-Rays confirmed that Jim had a slipped vertebra, *spondylolisthesis*, at the end of his

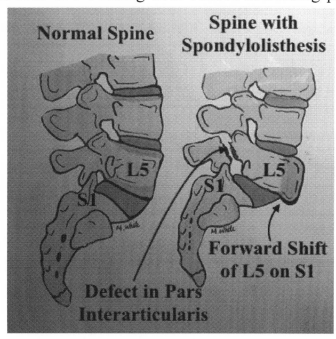

Side view a normal spine and one with a spondylolisthesis with the fifth lumbar vertebra slipped forward on the first sacral vertebra due to a fracture of the pars interarticularis

lumbar spine at L5-S1 causing his persistent back pain and irritating his right first sacral nerve root. He elected to have it stabilized with a spinal fusion. After four months, he was back at work part time. He returned full time to all his required duties as a mechanic at six months.

Spondylolisthesis is a Greek term for slippage of one vertebra on another. About five percent of patients with back pain have this condition.

The most common type is due to an excessive back bending injury to the lower lumbar spine where it meets the sacrum. Fractures occur where the vertebral body joins onto the back portion of the spine through the *pars interarticularis*.

This injury results in some back and leg pain, which may be transient in adolescents and young adults. It is commonly seen in gymnasts, football lineman and butterfly swimmers. If the pain persists, routine spine X-Rays and CT scans will show the slip and the fracture. Restriction from sports and bracing will usually resolve the pain and allow return to normal activities. Actual bony healing of the fracture defect is unlikely.

Degenerative Spondylolisthesis

This condition is due to collapse of the disc and arthritis of the facet joints that result in instability, usually between the fourth and fifth lumbar vertebrae. It is commonly seen in older women. They experience chronic low back pain and bilateral leg pain, which is worse with standing and bending and relieved with sitting and bed rest.

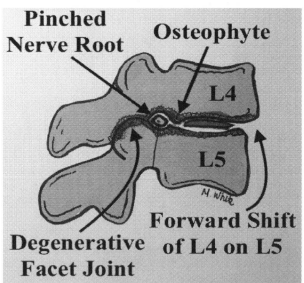

Degenerative Spondylolisthesis with Collapsed Disc

Conservative treatment with medication, bracing, physical therapy and injections may provide some relief. In many cases the patients become more symptomatic as their instability progresses and have greater difficulty in carrying out their activities of daily living.

Surgical fusion requires a few days in the hospital. The symptomatic level is exposed through several small incisions on each side of the lower back or through the midline to gain access to the intervertebral disc and nerve roots. A partial removal of the roof of the spine, a *laminectomy*, and *facetectomy* is necessary. After removal of the diseased disc, a

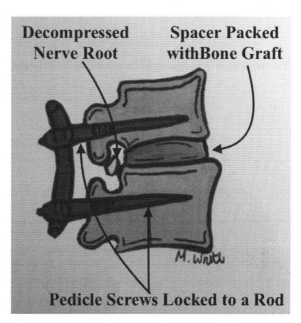

Decompressed Nerve Root

Spacer Packed withBone Graft

Pedicle Screws Locked to a Rod

Degenerative Spondylolisthesis after Correcting Slippage of Vertebrae and Fusion with Pedicle Screws and Spacer Packed with Bone Graft in Place of the Intervertebral Disc

plastic or metallic spacer filled with bone graft is inserted between the affected vertebrae to restore normal spacing and stability. In many cases the slip is also corrected. Strips of bone graft are placed over the transverse processes and remaining bone in the back of the spine to initiate fusion. In order to secure the spacer implant, screws are placed down the walls of the vertebrae, *pedicles*, and these are connected to rods. Over a period of four to six months, the bone in the spacer and along the transverse processes is expected to fuse the two vertebrae together.

Most patients following surgery get relief of their back and leg pain and are able to resume their normal daily activities. The surgeon must be careful in placing the spacer implant so as not to exert any pressure on the nerves roots.

Occasionally, following surgery, the patient may experience a short period of tingling, numbness and muscle weakness due to stretch of the exposed nerve roots. Blood clots, excessive bleeding and infection are rare complications.

Lumbar Spinal Stenosis

Harry, a sixty-year-old teacher, had difficulty with walking from his classroom to the parking lot, a distance of three blocks up a hill. It was not so much his back hurt as it was his legs. They started to ache as he walked and he had to stop and sit before continuing on. He noticed that if he leaned on the shopping cart in the supermarket he could walk without any leg pain. He could also ride an exercise bike without leg pain but had difficulty with the treadmill. He was very comfortable sitting at his desk. He saw his family doctor who suggested that he have x-rays and MRI of his lumbar spine. These studies showed that Harry had fairly advanced arthritis of his spine and pressure on the nerves going to his lower extremities. He had physical therapy and a series of steroid injections in his lower back which gave him some temporary relief. After several months he was referred to a spine surgeon who made a diagnosis of *lumbar spinal stenosis*. Harry had surgery to open up the spinal canal, *laminectomy*, to relieve the pressure on the affected nerves. He noted gradual improvement in his walking distance and relief of his leg pain.

Lumbar spinal stenosis is a very common spinal disorder that affects a number of older men and women. The spinal canal provides a channel for the spinal cord and nerves that travel to the extremities. The floor of the spinal canal is formed by the vertebrae and discs, the walls by pillars of bone called *pedicles* and the roof by the *laminae*.

As the patient's spinal arthritis worsens, the spinal canal becomes narrowed in diameter and reduced in cross sectional area due to the deformed and arthritic facet joints and collapse of the intervertebral disc. This results in compression of the spinal cord and nerves.

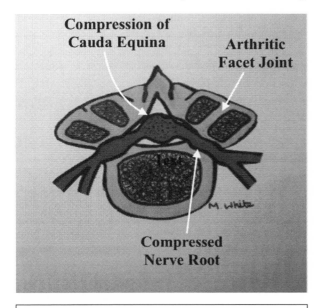

Illustration of Stenosis of Lumbar Spinal Canal Due to Arthritic Facets Causing Compression of the Cauda Equina and Nerve Roots

Imaging studies show degeneration of the discs, vertebral bodies and facet joints. Like Harry, patients complain of numbness and aching in their legs during walking. Sitting or lying on one's side with the hips and knees flexed will give them relief. As spinal stenosis progresses, patients lose their normal forward lumbar curve, lordosis, and become more bent over due to straightening of their lower spine. To compensate they may stand with their hips and knees flexed. Patients with diabetic neuropathy and those with peripheral vascular disease due to blockages in the arteries to their extremities will have similar complaints of aching, burning, and pain. Those with spinal stenosis can ride an exercise bicycle without difficulty in contrast to those with peripheral vascular disease who have difficulty due to the diminished blood supply to their muscles.

MRI, and in some cases, myelograms followed by CT scans, are necessary to determine the extent and location of the stenosis. These studies also guide the surgeon in treating the affected area. Fine needles placed in the muscles of the extremities, *EMG*, and nerve conduction tests, *NCT,* using electrical stimulation are used to differentiate spinal stenosis from diabetic nerve damage.

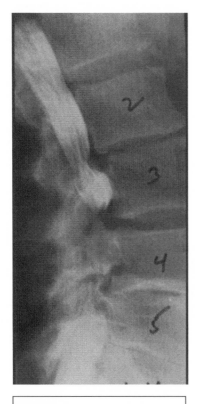

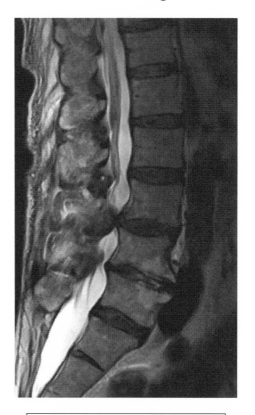

Myelogram – CT Scan of patient with spinal stenosis showing incomplete block at L2-L3 and complete block at L3-L4

MRI of patient with spinal stenosis showing blocks at L2-L3, L3-L4, and L4-L5

Early in the disease, NSAIDs and various types of land and water exercises may be helpful in reducing pain and maintaining posture and flexibility. As symptoms worsen, injections of cortisone into the space between the spinal covering*, dura*, and the spinal canal, *epidural space*, can be beneficial. In about a third of patients with lumbar spinal stenosis surgery is necessary. The most common areas involved are at the third, fourth, and fifth lumbar vertebrae.

Surgery consists of removing bone from the back of the spine, *laminectomy*, to open up the spinal canal. This procedure is called a *decompressive laminectomy.* Often portions of the arthritic facets are removed to open up the compromised passages*, foramen,* for the exiting nerve roots. If there is instability due to a forward or side slippage of the involved vertebrae or created during the decompression, a spinal fusion may be necessary. This can be done following the laminectomy by removing the discs and replacing them with metal or plastic implants called spacers loaded with bone grafts. The bone grafts are expected to, in time, result in a "welding together" of the affected vertebrae and restore stability. In order to keep these implants in place, screws are placed into the vertebral bodies and connected to metal rods. These instrumented fusions allow for safer mobilization and recovery than fusions done prior to the use of screws and rods.

Most patients leave the hospital a few days following the procedure. A brace may be prescribed by the surgeon to support the spine until the fusion is healed. Ambulation with a walker is started prior to leaving the hospital. Patients are shown how to transfer safely from bed to bathroom. Oral pain medication is usually necessary for a few weeks following surgery.

Swelling and pain in and around the operative area can be reduced by using a machine that delivers chilled water to neoprene sleeves that wrap around the lumbar area. Patients are encouraged to resume their activities of daily living during the first week or two after surgery.

It takes four to six months for the fusion to heal during which time one must not participate in lifting, heavy physical work or sports. Once the fusion is healed as determined by x-rays, these activities can be resumed gradually. The majority of patients undergoing surgery for lumbar spinal stenosis experience a good result and are able to resume a normal lifestyle including hobbies and sports. Patients who delay surgery and those with comorbidities such as diabetes and Parkinson's disease may not experience a good result. Infection is ten times more common in poorly controlled diabetics. Dysfunction of the nerves manipulated during surgery may occur. These nerves usually recover their full function. Failure to heal the fusion occurs in fewer than five percent and is common in smokers and those who are vitamin D deficient. Patients are cautioned to stop smoking and those with vitamin D deficiency are prescribed replacement therapy several weeks prior to their surgery.

Adult Spinal Deformity, Scoliosis

Jane, a sixty-three-year-old retired hospital administrator had been treated for scoliosis as a teenager with a plastic brace around her torso for several months. She married and had three children. In her early fifties she began to experience pain below her shoulder blades and in her lower back. She noted her clothes did not fit well because her right shoulder was higher than her left and her left hip appeared to be higher than her right. She was getting shorter.

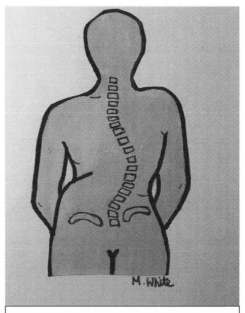

Common type of scoliosis: Note the high right shoulder, rotated and curved spine and uneven pelvic bones.

A year later she started having intermittent but disabling right hip, thigh and leg pain. She had to stop traveling to see her grandchildren. X-Rays of her spine showed she had a sixty-five-degree scoliosis with marked degeneration of the discs and bone in her spine. After trying several types of therapy, medications and injections, she had a corrective spinal fusion with rods and screws. She is now able to travel and is enjoying her grandkids.

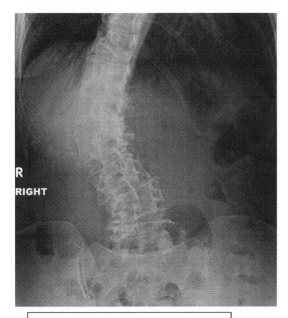

X-ray of patient with primary lumbar scoliosis

Scoliosis in adults can be the result of progression of their adolescent curves or due to degenerative changes and osteoporosis, which cause malalignment and instability of the spine as they age.

As with Jane, upper and lower back pain and muscle fatigue begin to occur in midlife. As the curvature of the spine increases, the shoulders and hips become more uneven and height is lost as the rib cage slowly descends down into the top of the pelvis. This causes a forward protuberance of the abdomen. Pain in the lower extremities due to irritation of the spinal nerves is common.

When one examines the spine with the patient standing there is usually a prominent upper (thoracic) or lower (lumbar) curve. In an attempt to align and balance the spine, the body compensates with secondary curves. Lower extremity pain occurs when the spinal nerves become stretched or compressed.

Standing X-Rays of the spine from head to pelvis are done to evaluate the degree and extent of the deformities. A check on the muscle strength, sensation and reflexes in the extremities is done. MRI and occasionally a myelogram and CT scan are done prior to surgery to detect areas of nerve root and spinal cord compression.

31

NSAID medications may be helpful early on. Pilates, Yoga, swimming and walking are helpful to keep fit and to maintain function. Injection of steroid medication into the spinal canal (epidural steroid) may give temporary relief of back and leg pain. Bracing may provide some relief.

Surgery to correct an adult spinal deformity should be undertaken with the understanding that one may experience one or more complications and that the process of recovery may take several

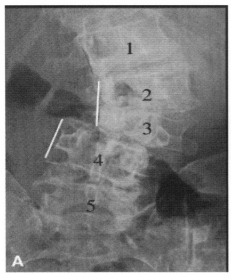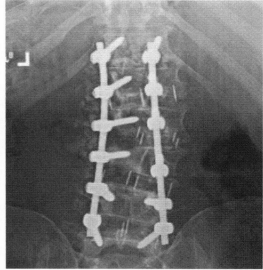

X-Rays of 55-year-old female with severe back and leg pain due to degenerative scoliosis with marked sideways slip of the third lumbar vertebra on the fourth lumbar vertebra. The scoliosis was corrected with interbody spacers and fixed with screws and rods.
Courtesy of Paul McAffee M.D.

months. Patients with significant cardiovascular and pulmonary issues and those with diabetes are more likely to have complications. The type of surgical procedure depends on the type of curve and its severity. If there are significant areas of nerve compression due to spinal stenosis, those must be treated.

The most common corrective surgery is performed through a long or several small back incisions. Bone is removed from areas of stenosis to provide more room for the compressed nerves. Discs are removed and metal or plastic spacers containing bone grafts are inserted to facilitate curve correction and to restore height. At times, these devices are inserted through small incisions placed through the side of the abdomen. Cutting and removal of parts of the vertebra in severe curves may be necessary. The spine is rebalanced and stabilized with multiple screws and rods. A combination of the patient's own bone, bone from a bone bank and various types of bone substitutes are added to the area prepared for fusion.

Blood collected prior to and during surgery from the patient or blood from the blood bank is often given during or shortly after surgery. Spinal cord function is monitored during the procedure. If the monitoring shows any abnormal signal changes, the surgical team is alerted and immediately proceeds to take corrective action to prevent a neurological deficit. A brace is worn until a fusion is confirmed by x-ray. Serious complications such as excessive blood loss, infection and permanent neurologic deficits are rare. Breakage of spinal fixation devices may be indicative of a failed fusion and may require further surgery.

Synovial Cyst
Synovial cysts, which are similar to the common ganglion cysts of the wrist, arise from the lining of the lumbar facet joints. These joints are arthritic and may be unstable. Because of this, the lining of the joint, *the synovium*, produces excess fluid, which is under pressure and forms a cyst filled with fluid. If the cyst compresses a nerve root or the dura, you may experience radicular pain in your lower extremity.

These cysts are often an incidental finding at surgery. They most commonly occur in the L4-L5 and L3- L4 facet joints. Removal of fluid from a cyst may be effective in relieving pressure on a nerve root. This is done with a needle under X-Ray control. However, there is a high recurrence rate and surgical treatment may be necessary.

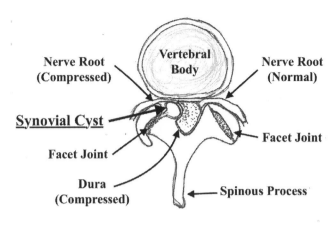

Synovial Cyst of the Spine
Viewed from Above

Nerve Root (Compressed)

Vertebral Body

Nerve Root (Normal)

Synovial Cyst

Facet Joint

Facet Joint

Dura (Compressed)

Spinous Process

Synovial cyst arising from a facet joint compressing the dura and a nerve root

Sacroiliac Joint Pain

Nancy, a fifty-five-year-old cyclist had a bad fall off her bicycle landing hard on her right buttock. Following her injury, she had difficulty walking, climbing stairs and turning in bed. She got very little relief from taking NSAIDs. After several weeks, she had imaging studies, which confirmed degenerative and arthritic changes in her SI joint. Physical therapy, stretching and manipulation of the joint did not provide any lasting relief. Anesthetic blocks plus cortisone gave her some relief for a few months. She subsequently had an SI joint fusion with metallic implants, which relieved her pain.

There are two SI joints, one on each side of your lower spine above your hips. These are the largest weight bearing joints of the body but only allow for a few degrees of motion. Because the SI joints are near the lower lumbar spine, SI joint pain is often confused with low back pain.

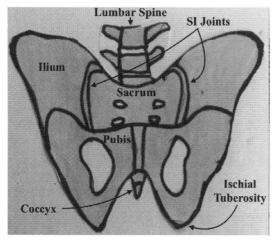

Frontal view of the Pelvis

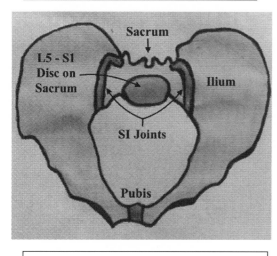

View from the top of the Pelvis showing the sacrum and SI joints

SI joint pain may result from injury as in Nancy's case, after pregnancy, spinal fusion and arthritis. Frequent complaints are pain with getting out of a chair, walking, climbing stairs, and turning over onto the affected side in bed. In some patients, pain from the inflamed SI joint will radiate from the buttocks into the thigh because of the close proximity of sensory nerves to the inflamed joint. Patients with Ankylosing Spondylitis, AS, will commonly complain of bilateral SI joint pain during the early onset of their progressive inflammatory disease.

Although imaging studies often show abnormalities, injections of long-acting local anesthetics and cortisone are needed to cinch the diagnosis. In the past five years, fusions of the SI joint using small incisions and implants has provided relief for a number of patients. SI joint dysfunction may affect 15-30% of patients with back and buttocks complaints.

Painful Coccyx, Tailbone

The coccyx is made up of five small bones joined together by very small discs and thin ligaments. In a thin patient, a fall on the buttocks can easily disrupt one or more of these connections. The patient will experience pain with sitting for brief periods of time due to the unstable joint. In time, most of these injuries heal but, in some, pain persists. Use of a polyurethane foam donut or pad with the back cut out may reduce pressure on the coccyx when seated. Injections of local anesthetics and cortisone may provide some relief. Occasionally surgical removal of part of the coccyx may be necessary.

Ischial Bursitis

When we sit, we bear a portion of our weight on the bottom areas of our pelvis called the ischial tuberosities. These structures are well padded with attached ligaments, tendons and bursa tissue. Treatment is directed at reducing pressure on the tuberosities. Occasionally a cortisone injection is necessary.

Chapter 5: Arthritis, Cancer of the Spine, Spine Infections and Spine Fractures

Arthritis of the Spine

The most common type of arthritis that affects the spine is osteoarthritis, which involves the facet joints and vertebrae. The intervertebral disc loses nuclear material as we age. Tears in the annulus fibrosus occur and the cushioning effect, the vertical height and the stability of the disc are reduced. We refer to this as *degenerative disc disease.* When degenerative disc disease occurs, arthritis of the facet joints and

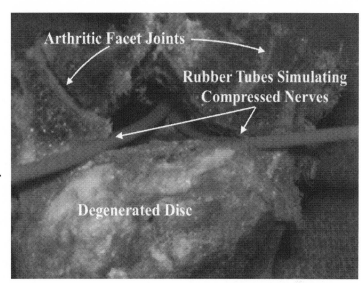

Cross-section of Cadaver Spine Showing Degeneratve Disc, Degenerative Arthritis of Facets, and Compression of Nerve Roots

surfaces of the vertebral bodies results. These structures form bone spurs, *osteophytes*. There is loss of height and reduction in the diameter of the spinal canal. This results in crowding and compression of the spinal cord and nerves, *spinal stenosis,* which is most commonly seen in the cervical and lumbar spine.

In addition, rheumatoid and other types of arthritis, such as that seen with inflammatory bowel diseases and psoriatic arthritis can strike the small and large joints of the spine causing a great deal of pain and disability. A condition called ankylosing spondylitis, *AS*, is a type of inflammatory arthritis that leads to progressive stiffness and fusion of the movable parts of the spine, the hips, sacroiliac joints and shoulders. AS makes one prone to spinal fractures due to lack of mobility and fragility of the vertebral bone. Patients with AS test positive for the HLA-B 27 antigen. There are several biologic immunotherapy medications being used to treat psoriatic arthritis, arthritis due to inflammatory bowel diseases and AS. Seukinumab® has recently been shown to benefit patients with AS.

Cancer of the Spine

Metastatic cancer frequently finds a home in the marrow of our long bones and spine. About 20,000 patients each year have cancer metastasic to their spine. Lung, breast, prostate and kidney are common sources of cancer metastasizing to the spine.

Ginny, age 55, came for consultation about persistent pain in her neck, worse at night and when she was inactive. Imaging studies showed two large bony lesions in her cervical vertebrae. She had had cancer of her breast treated several years ago. After a biopsy confirmed that these lesions were due to metastatic cancer from the breast, she underwent radiation and chemotherapy treatments that were successful.

Much less frequent are primary bone tumors that have their origin in bone. Some are benign bony growths like *osteochondromas*, and others are malignant and life-threatening such as *osteosarcoma*, bone cancer, and *chondrosarcoma*, cartilage cancer. These are very aggressive and invasive. These cancers present with deep unrelenting pain not related to movement or change in position. Pain at night is one of the hallmarks alerting the doctor to further explore this complaint. In addition to pain, the patient might experience progressive loss of motor and sensory function if the tumor causes pressure on adjacent nerves or the spinal cord. Fracture of the involved bone may occur without trauma.

Chordomas, a type of cartilage tumor, are malignant tumors of the spine. They commonly occur in the sacrum in the fifth to seventh decade of life in males. Bladder and rectal dysfunction may occur because of the invasion of the tumor around the sacral nerves, bladder and rectum, all of which are in close proximity. A combination of surgery and various types of radiation therapy are used to treat them. Imatinib®, a monoclonal antibody has been helpful in suppressing tumor growth.

Giant cell tumors are aggressive, destructive tumors that destroy bone in young females. Because of the vascularity of the tumor, preoperative blockage of the feeder blood vessels is done prior to surgical resection. Denosumab®, a monoclonal antibody has been used recently in treating patients with non-resectable tumors and in those with recurrence following surgery.

Our bone marrow is full of many types of cells, including red and white blood cells, lymphocytes, platelets, plasma cells, *osteoblasts*, bone forming cells, *osteoclasts*, bone destroying cells, and an array of *stem cells*. Stem cells are the source and generators of our specialized blood and tissue cells. When any of these cells multiply out of control, malignant cells are produced.

Multiple myeloma is a cancer of plasma cells, which originate in bone and is associated with pain and spontaneous fractures. The presence of abnormal antibodies in the blood and urine (Bence -Jones paraproteins) and a positive needle biopsy confirm the diagnosis. The treating physician should be suspicious of multiple myeloma in a patient with one or more compression fractures of the spine. MRI and CT scans are used to evaluate the location, type and extent of the disease. The abnormal myeloma proteins in the urine deposit casts which block kidney function and result in renal failure. Various types of chemotherapy are used to eradicate the cancerous plasma cells. If the patient has a good response to chemotherapy with a significant reduction of the abnormal plasma cells, *a stem cell transfer* using the patient's own bone marrow may result in a remission.

Susan, a 70-year-old avid golfer, who often walked 18 holes had persistent pain in her back that was worse at night and when she was inactive. Imaging studies showed two compression fractures in her thoracic and one in her lumbar spine. She underwent injections of bone cement into each fracture, *vertebroplasty,* but did not get any relief. She was given pain medication and was told she would need to "live with her pain." A few months later, additional tests were done including those for multiple myeloma which were positive. She began chemotherapy, which wiped out the majority of her malignant plasma cells and she subsequently had a successful stem cell transplant.

Various types of leukemia due to abnormal white cells, such as *myelocytic* and *lymphocytic*, may result in pain, anemia, fever and frequent infections due to a diseased and altered immune system. Chemotherapy and radiation are effective in suppressing leukemia. Fractures may occur in bone infiltrated with leukemia cells.

Infiltration of destructive cancer cells can cause sudden collapse of one or more vertebrae, instability of that segment of the spine and compression of the spinal cord. Depending on the location of the spinal cord compression, loss of function in the lower extremities, *paraplegia* or loss of function in both the upper and lower extremities, *quadriplegia* may result.

Metastatic lesions to the spine are best treated with chemotherapy and in some cases targeted immunotherapy. Metastatic cancer from the breast, lungs, prostate, kidney and gastrointestinal tract respond to radiation therapy. Surgery may be an option for patients expected to live a number of months and in relatively good health. Chemotherapy and radiation are often given to reduce tumor size prior to surgical intervention. Imaging studies are utilized to evaluate whether or not the tumor is amenable to surgical resection. Total resection of the diseased vertebra with preservation of the spinal cord and reconstruction with bone grafts and metallic fixation is feasible. Complications following this type of surgery may be serious and outcomes may be disappointing.

Spinal Infection

Henry, a healthy 30-year-old man, was recovering at home after undergoing a lumbar discectomy, when he had a sudden chill followed by a fever of 103 degrees. He also had increasing pain in the area of his back surgery. He reported this to his surgeon, who admitted him to the hospital. Blood tests and cultures confirmed that Henry was suffering from a postoperative infection. He received intravenous antibiotics, which were targeted to eradicate his type of infection, and he recovered.

Joe has adult onset diabetes; he had surgery for lumbar spinal stenosis. A few days later he felt poorly and had a low-grade fever with increasing pain in his operative area. He had received antibiotics before, during and for a day following surgery. Drainage from his incision was sent to the laboratory for culture, which grew out a "staph" bacteria. Antibiotics were restarted and he was returned to the operating room for drainage of a large abscess involving the tissues in the area of his surgery. After several weeks, the infection was brought under control and he returned home.

When Surgical Site infection occurs, we consider these factors:

1. Host resistance
2. Inoculum
3. Virulence of the bacteria
4. Presence of a foreign body

By "Host Resistance," we mean the ability of the body to resist infection. Our skin is covered and our intestines are filled with trillions of bacteria, our "biome." Every time we brush our teeth, we send bacteria into our blood stream, generally to no effect. If your

41

resistance is diminished by A.I.D.S, autoimmune diseases, diabetes or chronic use of steroids, you stand an increased chance of infection from surgery.

Your blood glucose needs to be in a suitable range before, during and after surgery. The rate of infection following spine surgery increases tenfold if your diabetes is in poor control.

The "Inoculum" is the number of bacteria that gets into the host. A tiny amount, such as what we may get from brushing our teeth, is unlikely to cause problems, but a huge amount is likely to overwhelm any host.

Surgeons do all they can to avoid this by extensively scrubbing their hands, wearing sterile clothing and gloves along with shields to protect their patients. Sterilizing instruments, using soaps and antiseptics to prepare the patient's skin, establishing a "sterile field" around the incision and managing airflow in the operating room are done to decrease infections.

Infection prevention is always on the minds of all operating room personnel who monitor each other on behalf of the patient. Likewise, patients need to carefully manage their own bodies by thoroughly washing with appropriate soaps before surgery. They should avoid skin cuts and scratches, especially on or near the body part having the surgery. For spine surgery, where implants are inserted into the body, we recommend getting dental work and regular dental cleaning well in advance of surgery.

The nose harbors bacteria that could infect the host. We recommend nasal swabs for MRSA, methicillin resistant staphylococcus aureus, a particularly difficult bacteria to eradicate. If MRSA is found in the nose, it can be treated before surgery with a specific antibiotic ointment.

"Virulence" describes the inherent aggressiveness of the bacteria. Highly virulent bacteria are very aggressive, so a smaller dose can cause an infection that may not occur with less virulent bacteria.

We live with low virulence bacteria all of the time, but when the bad ones, the highly virulent ones, come along we are apt to be in trouble.

A subtopic about virulence is the susceptibility of bacteria to antibiotics. Some, such as MRSA and others, are less susceptible to the usual antibiotics than others. They have become resistant over time from exposure to commonly used antibiotics.

Penicillin was the first antibiotic. Over time many bacteria became "penicillin resistant." Methicillin was developed to fight penicillin resistant bacteria, and the bacteria developed resistance to it, too. As we have regularly used the stronger, more-toxic-to-human antibiotics, some bacteria have become resistant to them, too.

We need to be judicious in our use of antibiotics since bacteria are constantly evolving and developing resistance. Our scientists are diligently developing new antibiotics, but it is a formidable task that we only make more challenging by overusing the ones that we have.

An important point for the short term is that surgeons use broad-spectrum antibiotics prophylactically beginning just before surgery and then for only a dose or two more. This helps to knock out any bacteria that may get into the surgical wound. That has been scientifically demonstrated to reduce the incidence of wound infection.

A "Foreign body" is anything in the body that we were not born with. It is well known that the presence of a foreign body, like a spinal implant, makes eradication of infection more difficult. Since spinal implants are used to stabilize the spine, they are usually retained when the wound is reopened and infected soft tissue is removed to treat infection.

Spinal infections may occur in patients with diabetes, those on long-term cortisone therapy, those with H.I.V. infection and in patients who are immunocompromised by diseases and medications that reduce a person's immunity. The most common complaints are neck and back pain which are constant and worse at night. There may be stiffness and reduced spinal motion. Typically, an infection is carried in the blood stream from another infected organ such as skin, lung, or kidney to the spine.

Blood tests, cultures of blood and drainage fluids, bone scans, CT scans and MRI are helpful in diagnosing and managing spinal infection.

It is important to **contact your physician** if you think you have an infection. **Do not start yourself on some random antibiotic** that you have saved in your medicine cabinet. Taking an antibiotic that will not be effective against the causative bacteria can interfere with laboratory cultures and delay treatment with the properly targeted antibiotic. Taking a random antibiotic will also convert one's biome from bacteria that are less resistant to antibiotics to ones that are more resistant, so if an infection occurs it will be more difficult to treat.

If an abscess develops in the space surrounding the spinal cord, *epidural abscess*, the patient may experience extremity weakness, numbness and lack of bladder and bowel control, *incontinence*. It is imperative to remove the epidural abscess to preserve spinal cord function. An infection that invades bone may result in progressive bone destruction and instability of the spine segment, which can also lead to permanent loss of spinal cord function and paralysis. Prolonged targeted antibiotics to combat sepsis, coupled with surgery to remove infected bone and to stabilize the involved spine segments are effective in the majority of those afflicted.

Compression Fractures.

When subjected to abnormal forces during a fall, the extremity bone or vertebra fails and a fracture occurs. Osteoporosis is most commonly seen in women around the time of menopause. Women with fair skin and blue eyes are especially prone to thinning of their bone, *osteopenia*, and softening of bone, *osteoporosis*. They often find out that they have osteoporosis only after they sustain a fracture.

Osteoporotic compression fractures are common in post-menopausal women after minor trauma. These so-called *fragility* fractures can be seen on a routine x-ray. However, a CT scan provides more detail. MRI helps distinguish old from new compression fractures and fractures associated with infection, tumors and cancer.

They are called "compression fractures" because the bone has been squashed or compressed. Think of a Styrofoam cube to which you apply some amount of weight. The weakest part of the vertebra is the vertebral body. Our spine supports us against gravity. Compression forces are directed more to the front of the spine causing a wedge shaped vertebral body deformity when a fracture occurs. Treatment may include bedrest, medication for pain and bracing. Rigid metal braces are poorly tolerated in contrast to lighter more flexible types. For fractures not responding to this treatment, *vertebroplasty* is an option. This procedure is done by placing a needle into the vertebral body and injecting bone cement to stabilize the fracture. A *kyphoplasty* elevates the compressed and fractured bone with a balloon device before fixing it with bone cement.

Kyphoplasty

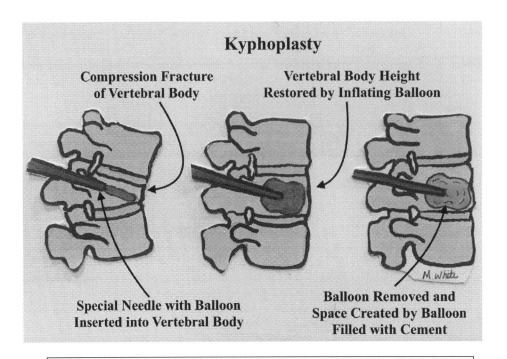

Compression Fracture of Vertebral Body

Vertebral Body Height Restored by Inflating Balloon

M White

Special Needle with Balloon Inserted into Vertebral Body

Balloon Removed and Space Created by Balloon Filled with Cement

Balloon Kyphoplasty with Cement for Compression Fracture

Patients with multiple compression fractures develop a bent over posture referred to as a dowager's hump. In order to stand erect and maintain their posture they extend their neck and flex their hips and knees for balance. They also lose vertical height and develop a protrusion of their abdomen making them appear obese.

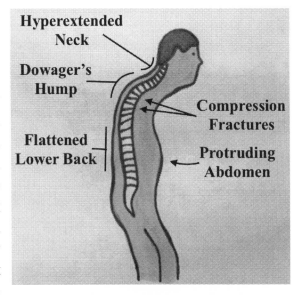

Hyperextended Neck

Dowager's Hump

Flattened Lower Back

Compression Fractures

Protruding Abdomen

Patient with dowager's hump due to compression fractures

Due to a lack of spine mobility, back and neck spine fractures occur commonly with low impact trauma in patients with Ankylosing Spondylitis, AS. These fractures often displace and move causing pressure on the spinal cord and nerve roots which can result in paralysis. Surgery is needed to realign and stabilize these fractures in order to get the patient out of bed and prevent further damage to the spinal cord.

Older patients who are subjected to high impact trauma, such as may occur in a motor vehicle accident, may suffer fractures as well as failure of spinal stability, *dislocations*, of the spine. These may lead to complete or incomplete motor paralysis and sensory loss in the extremities with loss of bowel and bladder control.

Chapter 6: Complications of Spine Surgery

In this chapter, we will address the complications that keep surgeons awake at night worrying about their patients and some factors that can have an effect on the complication rate.

No surgeon thinks that a surgical procedure on him or herself is a minor procedure and no experienced surgeon thinks that any procedure is not potentially subject to complications. It is all a matter of degree, and we have seen plenty.

Neurologic Complications

Injuries to the spinal cord during spine surgery are very rare. The use of spinal cord monitoring during surgery alerts the surgical team to a potential neurologic deficit so they can take corrective measures. These may require increasing the blood pressure to better supply blood to the spinal cord, release tension on instrumentation and implants and check for compression on the spinal cord and nerve roots at the sites of corrective procedures. Tears of the dura are not uncommon and need watertight repair. Occasionally a nerve will be stretched or traumatized during surgery, but these generally recover over time.

Failure to Heal Your Fusion

Spinal fusion is a joining together of two or more spine segments. Surgeons create the situation for fusions to occur but the body has to grow the bones together. With modern instrumentation and various types of bone grafts and bone enhancing products, there is a very high rate of spine fusion, but in 5-7% of patients there is a failure of those fusions to occur. Failed fusion is more common when several spine levels are joined together in older adults with spinal deformity. These failed fusions are often painful and associated with breakage of spinal implants. Some of these fusions can be salvaged non-surgically by using external electrical devices to stimulate bone union. Some require revision surgery with new grafts and implants.

Excessive Bleeding and Hematomas

Bleeding during surgery is expected. Rapid loss of blood may occur when working on the front of the lumbar spine in close proximity to the iliac veins and their branches. Some bleeding after surgery is expected, but it should be reasonable and proportionate to the amount and type of surgery performed.

For some spine procedures, your surgeon is likely to have blood prepared to transfuse if necessary. There are potential complications from transfusion, specifically cross match issues causing a reaction, and transmission of diseases like hepatitis and A.I.D.S. Fortunately transfusion issues are very uncommon.

Due to preventative screening and modern matching techniques, during our many years of surgery with transfusing blood fairly often, we **rarely** saw any transfusion complications.

Transfusions are needed less often today than in the past. A cell saver machine is used to collect your own blood, wash it and return it to you during surgery. Various chemical agents added to the circulating blood and surgical site reduce bleeding by blocking the body's substances that cause clot breakdown.

You can build up your red cell volume with medications before surgery. Donating your own blood is another option that is used fairly often. However, this somewhat depletes your red cell level going into surgery. The complication rate of using blood donated by others is no higher than that of using your own.

Although it may be hard to do, you need to stop your anti-inflammatory medications such as ibuprofen at least a week to ten days before surgery. These medications affect your platelet function and can result in poor clotting and persistent oozing. If you are on anticoagulants, blood thinners, you will have to stop them. It takes a few days for their effect to wear off.   Before stopping your anticoagulants, you must consult the physician who prescribed them. Sometimes a short acting anticoagulant, such as heparin, can be used prior to surgery.

"Hematoma" is another result of excessive bleeding and can be in the form of liquid or clotted blood. Blood often leaks out through the incision. If the incision is watertight, however, the blood is trapped inside. To prevent hematoma formation, drain tubes connected to suction bulbs are commonly used in spine surgery.

An epidural hematoma can cause serious compression of the spinal cord and nerve roots. These hematomas can cause progressive neurologic deficits. They demand immediate return to surgery to evacuate them and relieve the pressure on the neural structures.

DVT (Deep Vein Thrombosis)

Deep vein thrombosis is fairly uncommon after most surgeries on the spine. When a clot occurs in a pelvic or extremity vein, it can cause pain and significant swelling of the extremity. Ultrasound studies confirm the presence and location of the clot usually in a deep vein in the pelvis or extremity. The clot can often be removed by a skilled vascular surgeon. Anticoagulants like heparin are used to treat and prevent DVTs. Because of the fear of bleeding around the dura, anticoagulants are not an option. Filter barriers are placed in the vena cava, the major abdominal vein, to block clots from going to the lungs.

Pulmonary embolus, *PE*, occurs when a clot of blood breaks loose and lodges in the lung. This impairs pulmonary blood flow, which impairs the transfer of oxygen into the blood stream, a serious and sometimes fatal condition. Initial symptoms include sudden-onset chest pain, shortness of breath, and coughing, sometimes producing blood. A *DVT* above the knee is much more likely than one below the knee to be fatal by breaking off and going to the lungs causing a pulmonary embolus. A residual clot may cause chronic pain and swelling of the extremity.

There are many causes of DVT but being stuck in bed following surgery may significantly increase one's risk. After surgery, you are in a hypercoagulable state, i.e. more prone to your blood clotting. DVT can occur in the arms as well as the legs.

Efforts to prevent DVT begin in the operating room with compression stockings and devices that milk the fluid from the foot upward. Patients are encouraged to work their feet up and down to activate their "calf pump." This action is provided by contracting the calf muscles, which squeeze blood out of the veins and pumps it upward. Getting out of bed and walking is necessary to help prevent clots from forming. When in bed or a chair, your legs need to be elevated to encourage blood and fluid to move toward the trunk as opposed to pooling in your legs.

Clinical examination may be unreliable. If there is any question of a DVT, an ultrasound needs to be done.

Pulmonary Conditions

Aside from pulmonary embolus, other pulmonary problems include *atelectasis* and *pneumonia*. Atelectasis is incomplete filling of the tiny air sacs in the lungs that occurs when the chest is not regularly and fully expanded.

This can allow fluids to collect and stagnate resulting in pneumonia.

You are encouraged to take deep breaths, use the breathing devices provided to you, sit up in a chair as soon as possible and walk as much as you can.

It's all about taking really deep breaths.

Pneumonia is well known to everyone and results when bacteria infect the lungs.

Bladder Problems

Anesthesia and narcotic painkillers make it hard for most people to urinate after surgery. Putting an older man with a slightly enlarged prostate in bed where he cannot stand up to void and giving him narcotics is a surefire recipe for urinary retention.

If straining, sitting up, running water and other magic do not work, a catheter will have to be inserted to allow urine to flow.

After a few hours or days when the patient has been getting up and walking and pain medications have been reduced, the problem usually resolves.

Easy solution, huh?

Yes, unless one develops a bladder infection from an indwelling catheter, one of the most common causes of hospital-acquired infection. Thus, intermittent catherization is less convenient but generally safer.

Bedsores (Decubitus Ulcers)

The skin can tolerate only a very few hours of direct pressure without breaking down. If you sit in a chair too long you'll notice that your rear end begins to hurt or tingle. If your sensation is impaired from drugs and you are stuck in bed, you're at high risk for a bedsore. You have to get up or change positions to relieve the pressure so blood can nourish the skin and soft tissues.

Bony prominences such as the sacrum, the lower end of the spine just above the tailbone, the sides of the hips, and the backs of the heels are especially prone to ulcerate. As with everything else, the skin is older people is less resistant to breakdown.

As always, prevention is the best treatment. You should move as much as you can.

If you feel something stinging on your buttocks, your heel or anywhere, and you cannot move to unload that spot, notify your nurse. The cushions under your legs to protect your heels and the mattress automatically inflating and deflating in different spots may be annoying but that they are necessary to help you avoid what could become a major problem.

A Word of Encouragement

If you have ever wondered why surgeons are extremely uncomfortable about having surgery themselves, reading the scary information above should explain why.

We know too much about complications.

Fortunately, the infection rate in our hospitals is generally less than 2%.

There is never "no chance" of something going wrong despite all of our best efforts, but the odds are overwhelmingly in your favor.

Chapter 7: What to Expect from Your Surgery, "Outcomes"

Everyone having surgery wants a good outcome.

How do we judge a good outcome? You can simply ask the following questions:

Is your pain relieved or better?

Can you do your usual daily activities without restriction?

Can you participate in hobbies and sports without limitation?

Would I make the decision to have surgery again for the same problem?

When you see your physician, he or she will ask what degree of pain you are experiencing on a scale of one to ten, ten being the worst. You should try to pick a number that represents the average degree of pain you are experiencing. While sitting in the waiting room or lying on the examination table you might have little or no pain. During the physical examination, if the doctor touches or stresses a painful area let him or her know this is where your usual pain is located.

Beside pain, your physician wants to know how limited you are in carrying out your activities of daily living, work obligations, hobbies and sports. Injuries and disorders of the musculoskeletal system often result in significant functional deficits. In order to objectively evaluate the results of treatment, "standardized functional outcomes measures" are used. There are several commonly used outcome measures for each anatomical body area. These assessment tools are often included in the forms you fill out before and after surgery. Your physical and occupational therapist will record measurements of your physical and functional status as you progress through your pre or post-operative rehabilitation program.

John undergoes surgery for a slipped vertebra, spondylolisthesis, in his low back. Initially he will have difficulty with getting in and out of bed, dressing, walking, and going up and down stairs. As he progresses in rehab these activities of daily living will be easier and should return to normal. His surgeon will be rating John's mobility, strength and gait. His therapist will be charting his functional improvement following each therapy session.

Outcomes assessments are used to evaluate the effectiveness of various treatments. Treatments which result in poor or less than satisfactory outcomes are discarded. Insurance companies and Medicare pay close attention to data generated from outcomes assessments. Decisions to provide coverage for a novel procedure or device are dependent on peer reviewed, scientific journal articles containing statistically significant, objective outcome data.

Glossary

Anterior, Ventral, the front of the spine

Posterior, Dorsal, the back view of the spine

Lateral, the side view of the spine

Cranial, Superior, toward the head

Caudal, Inferior, toward the tail

Flexion, forward bending of the spine

Extension, backward bending of the spine

Rotation, turning of the spine

Lateral, bending to the side

Lordosis, normal forward curve of the cervical and lumbar spine

Kyphosis, normal backward curve of the thoracic spine

Scoliosis, combination of lateral bending and rotation of the spine

Spondylolistheses, forward slip of one vertebra upon another

Vertebral body, a cylindrical bone which forms the base of the spinal canal

Pedicles, lateral projections extending from the back of the vertebral body

Laminae, plates of bone covering the back of the spinal canal

Spinous process, projections of bone you can feel on your back

Superior and Inferior facets, allow for coupling of one vertebra to the other

Transverse process, provide for muscle attachments

Spinal Canal, bony canal that provides protection for the spinal cord and nerves

Intervertebral Disc, composed of nuclear gel-like material, the nucleus pulposus, surrounded by interlacing fibers of the annulus fibrosus with attachments to the vertebral bodies

Sacrum, five vertebra all joined together without discs

Coccyx, five, small, tail-like vertebrae

Sacroiliac Joint, large joints between the sacrum and the iliac bones of the pelvis

Spinal Cord, starts at the base of the brain and stops at the first lumbar vertebra, carries motor and sensory nerves to the extremities and trunk

Spinal Nerve Roots, exit through openings in spine, **foramen,** to supply innervation to muscle, skin, ligaments and joints

Cauda Equina, collection of nerve roots beginning at the bottom of the spinal cord in lumbar spine

Dura, thick protective covering over brain and spinal cord

Epidural, just external to the outer surface of the dura

Spinal fusion, a joining together of one spine segment to another with bone

Osteotomy, cutting of bone

Stabilization, to rebalance and "shore-up"

Implant, a replacement part, for example a disc replacement

Instrumentation, used to hold correction and stabilize the spine, for example pedicle screws coupled with rods

NSAIDs, Non- steroidal anti-inflammatories drugs

CT Scans, Computerized tomography, a type of x-ray that allow three-dimensional (3D) visualization of the spine

MRI, Magnetic Radiographic Imaging uses high strength electromagnets rather than radiation to image the spine.

DEXA, Dual Energy X-ray Absorption scan uses low dose X-ray beams to measure bone density.

EMG, **E**lectro**m**yography, is used to detect abnormal nerve and muscle function by sampling the response of various muscles and nerves to signals from the brain.

NCT, **N**erve **C**onduction **T**ests uses electrical stimulation to evaluate whether or not the nerve is transmitting signals properly and at what speed.

SSEP, Somatosensory Evoked Potentials, monitor the sensory function of the spinal cord and nerves to electrical stimulation during surgery.

MEP, Motor Evoked Potentials, measure the motor function of the spinal cord and nerves to electrical stimulation during surgery.

Acknowledgements

We cannot possibly thank everyone who helped and inspired us along the way. Our wives have steadfastly stood beside us. They have been there for us on many family occasions when we were caring for patients. We thank them from the bottom of our hearts. Without them, our careers and our lives outside of work would have been meaningless.

We owe a profound thanks to those who helped educate us: our teachers in grammar school, high school, university, and medical school, and the professors and support staff in our orthopaedic training programs who gave so much of themselves to help us learn and understand our profession.

Special thanks go to novelist and acclaimed Professor of Orthopaedic Surgery Laurence Dahners, M.D. for his recommendations and assistance in publishing this book. Also, to Madeline White, a junior premedical student at Virginia Tech, Dick's grandniece, for her meaningful illustrations.

We deeply appreciate our volunteer readers who worked diligently to help make this book more readable, Ed Hearn, Diane Torgerson, Al Wordsworth, John Roper, Charlotte Hackman and Martin Myerson. A very special thanks to Marie Gillis for doing the final edits and proofing. Any errors you may find are ours, but without our readers there would be many more.

Finally, we are most appreciative to you for reading this work. As it is the second in a series, we would like to hear from you about what you like and do not like, so we can try to improve with each book.

Posting a candid review on Amazon would be most appreciated.

About the Authors

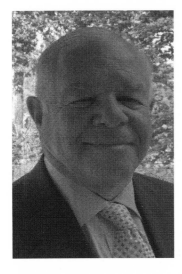

Richard J. Nasca, M.D. was born in Elmira NY and is a graduate of Georgetown College and Georgetown Medical School. He completed his internship at the Hospital of the University of Pennsylvania and postgraduate training in Surgery and Orthopaedics at Duke University and Affiliated Hospitals.

Dr. Nasca served as Chief of the Amputee and Hand Services at the Philadelphia Naval Hospital caring for Vietnam casualties. He held teaching appointments in Orthopaedic Surgery at the University of Arkansas School of Medicine and the University of Alabama School of Medicine. During his time in practice, he specialized in caring for patients with spine deformities, injuries and disorders.

He has been married to Carol T. Smith, R.N. for fifty-two years and has three children and one granddaughter. Dr. Nasca lives in Wilmington N.C. He is a volunteer physician at local medical clinics, on Advisory Boards at the College of Health and Human Services at University of North Carolina at Wilmington and has published six books, several book chapters and seventy peer reviewed scientific articles.

Dr. Nasca works in the soup kitchen and does fund raising for the Good Shepherd Center, is involved with the First Tee program, and is a certified Master Gardener. He enjoys golf, gardening, swimming and travelling.

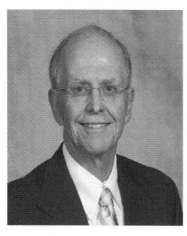 **James D. Hundley, M.D.** is a graduate of the University of the North Carolina School of Medicine and the Orthopaedic Surgery Residency Program of UNC Hospitals. After completing his orthopaedic training, he served as an orthopaedic surgeon in the U.S. Air Force for two years before joining an orthopaedic group practice in Wilmington, N.C.

His primary medical interests were in sports medicine where he was a university team physician for over twenty years and adult reconstruction (primarily hip and knee replacement surgery). Retired from medical practice, he continues to operate OrthopaedicLIST.com, a resource for orthopaedic surgeons founded in 2003.

Hundley's peers in orthopaedic surgery, the UNC School of Medicine, UNC Wilmington, his community, and his state have recognized him for his efforts. He continues to serve on non-profit boards and a foundation focused on community health.

His writings include multiple scientific papers published in medical journals, numerous magazine articles, and two blogs: www.agingdocs.com and http://www.orthopaediclist.com/blog.

Hundley and his wife, to whom he has been happily married for fifty years, have three children and five beautiful granddaughters. His other interests include golf, fishing, and reading.

Reviewers Comments

The book is clear and informative and will be helpful to many facing surgery. I especially like the case studies, which add a human touch to the science/medicine. —John R.

Where was **My Back Hurts** *in 2015 when I was struggling with my painful back? I was having back pains and finding little help. Finally, I went to a Chiropractor who took X-rays and found compression fractures. With this information, I had a bone density test made that showed low bone density. Kyphoplasty was a great help with the bone fractures! I wish I had access to* **My Back Hurts** *back then. My life and my back would have gotten much better a lot faster. Do yourself a huge favor if you have back issues and read* **My Back Hurts**. --Al W.

I think this is excellent for laymen. I just read most of it, looking for information regarding my own problems and I find it very easy to read and understand. The progression of thoughts and ideas follow well and easily make sense. Illustrations are nicely and clearly done. Such a good help for people with these problems. Especially when they come away from an appointment and don't really understand the information or words. --Diane T.

Both **My Hip Hurts** *and* **My Back Hurts** *are extremely well done. Having owned a printing business for 32 years, I like the size of the book, the type style used, the color of inks on the front and the paper selection. It's all user friendly. For the average person just looking to understand their condition more completely, you've 'hit the nail on the head.* --Ed H.

This is an important reference especially for seniors and anyone who experiences back pain... and who doesn't??
--Charlotte H

Made in the USA
Monee, IL
07 August 2021